THE LACTO-VEGETARIAN DIET COOKBOOK FOR BEGINNERS

Delicious Dishes: Simple meal plan with Easy Recipes to Help you living a healthy Life

Norval Ernser

Copyright

Table of Contents

Introduction

In a quaint little town nestled between rolling hills and lush meadows, there lived a young woman named Eliza. Eliza possessed a unique gift that set her apart from others in her community. She had an extraordinary ability to concoct the most delectable dishes merely by reading a recipe book. Her favorite tome? "The Lacto-Vegetarian Diet Cookbook for Beginners."

Eliza's humble kitchen was her sanctuary, adorned with shelves brimming with cookbooks of all shapes and sizes. However, it was the Lacto-Vegetarian cookbook that held a special place in her heart. Its pages were well-worn and splattered with ingredients from countless experiments.

One crisp morning, as the sun painted the sky in hues of pink and gold, Eliza awoke with an insatiable craving to create something extraordinary. With a determined gleam in her eye, she reached for her trusted cookbook. Flipping through its pages, she paused at a recipe titled "Creamy Spinach and Mushroom Stuffed Shells."

With the precision of a seasoned chef, Eliza gathered the necessary ingredients from her pantry and refrigerator. Fresh spinach, plump mushrooms, creamy ricotta cheese, and al dente pasta shells were carefully laid out on her worn wooden countertop.

Following the instructions meticulously, Eliza sautéed the spinach and mushrooms until they were tender and fragrant. In a separate bowl, she combined the ricotta cheese with a hint of nutmeg, creating a velvety-smooth filling. With deft hands, she stuffed each pasta shell with the luscious mixture, arranging them in a baking dish.

As the stuffed shells baked in the oven, filling her kitchen with mouthwatering aromas, Eliza couldn't help but smile with anticipation. She knew that her creation would be nothing short of spectacular.

When the timer chimed, signaling that her masterpiece was ready, Eliza carefully removed the baking dish from the oven. The shells emerged golden brown and bubbling, their savory scent wafting through the air.

With eager hands, Eliza plated the stuffed shells, garnishing them with a sprinkle of fresh herbs for a burst of color and flavor. With each bite, she savored the creamy richness of the filling, the earthy notes of the spinach and mushrooms dancing on her palate.

Word of Eliza's culinary prowess spread like wildfire throughout the town, attracting curious food enthusiasts from far and wide. Yet, for Eliza, the true joy lay not in the praise she received, but in the simple act of bringing people together through the power of food.

And so, armed with her beloved cookbook and boundless creativity, Eliza continued to delight and inspire all who had the pleasure of tasting her creations, one delicious dish at a time.

Introduction

Welcome to "The Lacto-Vegetarian Diet Cookbook for Beginners"! We're thrilled to embark on this culinary journey with you, introducing you to the vibrant and flavorful world of lacto-vegetarian cuisine. Whether you're new to the lacto-vegetarian lifestyle or simply looking for fresh inspiration in the kitchen, this cookbook is crafted to guide you through simple yet delicious recipes that promote both health and sustainability.

Understanding the Lacto-Vegetarian Diet

At its core, the lacto-vegetarian diet is centered around plant-based foods while incorporating dairy products such as milk, cheese, and yogurt. By excluding meat, poultry, fish, and eggs, lacto-vegetarians embrace a diet rich in fruits, vegetables, whole grains, legumes, nuts, and seeds. This dietary choice not only offers a wide array of nutrients but also aligns with ethical and environmental values by reducing reliance on animal products.

Benefits of Lacto-Vegetarianism

Embracing a lacto-vegetarian lifestyle can bring about a multitude of benefits, both for your personal well-being and for the planet. From improved heart health and weight management to reduced environmental impact and animal welfare, the advantages of choosing plant-based meals are far-reaching and compelling.

Tips for Success on the Lacto-Vegetarian Diet

Transitioning to a lacto-vegetarian diet may seem daunting at first, but with the right approach, it can be an enjoyable and sustainable journey. Throughout this cookbook, we'll share practical tips and strategies to help you navigate grocery shopping, meal planning, and cooking with confidence. Whether you're craving comforting classics or adventurous new flavors, we've got you covered with recipes that are both accessible and enticing.

Get ready to embark on a delicious culinary adventure that celebrates the abundance of plant-based ingredients and the joy of mindful eating. Let's dive in and discover the endless possibilities of the lacto-vegetarian diet together!

Understanding the Lacto-Vegetarian Diet

The lacto-vegetarian diet is a plant-based eating plan that excludes meat, poultry, fish, and eggs, but includes dairy products like milk, cheese, and yogurt. This dietary choice is often motivated by health reasons, ethical considerations, or a desire for more sustainable food practices.

Health Benefits

Lacto-vegetarianism offers numerous health benefits. By focusing on plant-based foods, individuals can reduce their intake of saturated fats and cholesterol, which are often found in animal products. This can lead to lower risks of heart disease, high blood pressure, and certain types of cancer. Additionally, plant-based diets are rich in fiber, vitamins, and antioxidants, which are essential for overall health and well-being.

Ethical and Environmental Considerations

Many people choose a lacto-vegetarian diet due to concerns about animal welfare and environmental sustainability. By avoiding meat and other animal products, individuals can reduce their impact on the environment, including greenhouse gas emissions, water usage, and deforestation associated with animal agriculture.

Nutritional Considerations

While a lacto-vegetarian diet can be nutritious, it's important to ensure that you're getting all the essential nutrients your body needs. This includes protein, iron, calcium, vitamin B12, and omega-3 fatty acids, which are commonly found in animal products. Fortunately, these nutrients can be obtained from plant-based sources and fortified foods, ensuring a well-rounded and balanced diet.

Making the Transition

Transitioning to a lacto-vegetarian diet can be a gradual process. It's helpful to start by incorporating more plant-based foods into your meals and experimenting with new recipes. Planning balanced meals and snacks, as well as seeking guidance from a healthcare professional or nutritionist, can also help ensure that you're meeting your nutritional needs.

Understanding the lacto-vegetarian diet is the first step towards embracing a more plant-based lifestyle. Whether you're motivated by health, ethics, or the environment, this dietary choice can have a positive impact on your well-being and the world around you. This cookbook is designed to inspire and support you on your lacto-vegetarian journey, providing delicious and nutritious recipes that will delight your taste buds and nourish your body.

Benefits of Lacto-Vegetarianism

Embracing a lacto-vegetarian lifestyle offers a multitude of benefits that extend beyond personal health to encompass ethical considerations and environmental sustainability. By choosing to focus on plant-based foods while incorporating dairy products, individuals can experience positive outcomes for themselves and the world around them.

Health Benefits

One of the primary benefits of adopting a lacto-vegetarian diet is its potential to improve overall health and well-being. Research suggests that plant-based diets can lower the risk of chronic diseases such as heart disease, diabetes, and certain types of cancer. By reducing intake of saturated fats and cholesterol found in animal products, while increasing consumption of fruits, vegetables, whole grains, and legumes, individuals can enjoy better cardiovascular health, improved weight management, and enhanced longevity.

Ethical Considerations

Lacto-vegetarianism aligns with ethical principles centered on compassion and respect for all living beings. By abstaining from the consumption of meat, individuals contribute to the reduction of animal suffering and exploitation in the food industry. This dietary choice reflects a conscious decision to promote kindness and empathy towards animals, acknowledging their intrinsic value and right to a life free from harm.

Environmental Sustainability

The environmental impact of food production is a growing concern in today's world. Animal agriculture is associated with significant greenhouse gas emissions, water usage, deforestation, and pollution. By reducing reliance on meat and dairy products, lacto-vegetarians can lessen their ecological footprint and contribute to a more sustainable food system. Choosing plant-based foods supports conservation efforts, reduces pressure on natural resources, and helps mitigate climate change.

Personal Empowerment

Adopting a lacto-vegetarian diet empowers individuals to take control of their health and make informed choices about the foods they consume. By embracing a diverse array of plant-based ingredients, individuals can explore new flavors, textures, and culinary traditions, expanding their palate and culinary repertoire. This dietary flexibility fosters creativity in the kitchen and encourages a deeper appreciation for the abundance of nature's bounty.

The benefits of lacto-vegetarianism extend far beyond personal health to encompass ethical considerations, environmental sustainability, and personal empowerment. By embracing a diet rich in plant-based foods while incorporating dairy products, individuals can nourish their bodies, cultivate compassion towards animals, and contribute to a healthier planet for future generations. This cookbook is designed to celebrate the myriad benefits of lacto-vegetarianism, offering delicious and nutritious recipes that reflect the diversity and vibrancy of plant-based eating.

Tips for Success on the Lacto-Vegetarian Diet

Transitioning to a lacto-vegetarian diet can be an exciting and rewarding journey towards improved health, ethical living, and environmental sustainability. To help you navigate this dietary transition successfully, we've compiled a list of practical tips and strategies to support you every step of the way.

1. Educate Yourself

Start by familiarizing yourself with the principles and guidelines of the lacto-vegetarian diet. Learn about the foods you can eat, including fruits, vegetables, grains, legumes, nuts, seeds, and dairy products. Understanding the nutritional benefits of plant-based foods will help you make informed choices and ensure you're meeting your dietary needs.

2. Plan Balanced Meals

Meal planning is essential for maintaining a balanced and nutritious diet. Aim to include a variety of foods in each meal, including sources of protein, carbohydrates, healthy fats, vitamins, and minerals. Experiment with different ingredients and recipes to keep your meals interesting and satisfying.

3. Stock Up on Staples

Keep your kitchen stocked with essential pantry staples for lacto-vegetarian cooking, such as grains (rice, quinoa, oats), legumes (beans, lentils, chickpeas), nuts, seeds, herbs, spices, and cooking oils. Having these ingredients on hand will make it easier to whip up delicious and nutritious meals at home.

4. Explore New Flavors

Embrace the diversity of plant-based cuisine by exploring new flavors, ingredients, and culinary traditions. Incorporate a variety of fruits, vegetables, herbs, and spices into your meals to add depth and complexity to your dishes. Don't be afraid to experiment with different cooking techniques and flavor combinations to find what works best for you.

5. Stay Mindful of Nutritional Needs

While a lacto-vegetarian diet can be healthy and nutritious, it's important to pay attention to your nutritional needs and ensure you're getting all the essential nutrients your body requires. Focus on incorporating a wide range of nutrient-dense foods into your diet, including sources of protein, iron, calcium, vitamin B12, and omega-3 fatty acids.

6. Be Prepared When Dining Out

Eating out as a lacto-vegetarian doesn't have to be challenging. Research restaurants in your area that offer vegetarian and dairy-friendly options, and don't hesitate to ask about menu substitutions or modifications to accommodate your dietary preferences. When in doubt, choose dishes that feature plenty of vegetables, grains, and dairy alternatives.

7. Listen to Your Body

Above all, listen to your body and honor its signals. Pay attention to how different foods make you feel and adjust your diet accordingly. If you're feeling low on energy or experiencing any discomfort, consider consulting with a healthcare professional or registered dietitian for personalized guidance and support.

By following these tips for success on the lacto-vegetarian diet, you'll be well-equipped to embrace a plant-based lifestyle with confidence and enthusiasm. Whether you're motivated by health, ethics, or the environment, making the switch to a lacto-vegetarian diet can have a positive impact on your well-being and the world around you. So, roll up your sleeves, sharpen your knives, and get ready to embark on a delicious and fulfilling culinary adventure!

Chapter 1: Breakfast Delights

Start your day off on the right foot with these delicious lacto-vegetarian breakfast recipes that are both satisfying and nutritious. From hearty smoothie bowls to savory omelettes, these morning meals are sure to energize you and set a positive tone for the day ahead.

1. Creamy Berry Smoothie Bowl

Indulge in a refreshing and satisfying breakfast with this creamy berry smoothie bowl. Packed with antioxidants, vitamins, and minerals, this vibrant dish is as nutritious as it is delicious. Simply blend together a combination of frozen berries, banana, Greek yogurt, and a splash of milk until smooth and creamy. Pour the smoothie into a bowl and top it with your favorite toppings, such as granola, sliced fruit, nuts, and seeds, for added crunch and flavor.

2. Veggie Omelette with Feta Cheese

Start your day with a protein-packed veggie omelette that's bursting with flavor. Whisk together eggs with a splash of milk and season with salt and pepper. Heat a non-stick skillet over medium heat and pour in the egg mixture. As the eggs begin to set, add your favorite vegetables, such as spinach, bell peppers, tomatoes, and onions, along with crumbled feta cheese. Once the omelette is cooked through, fold it in half and serve hot with a side of whole grain toast or fresh fruit.

3. Banana Walnut Pancakes

Treat yourself to a stack of fluffy banana walnut pancakes that are sure to delight your taste buds. In a mixing bowl, combine flour, baking powder, salt, mashed banana, milk, and a splash of vanilla extract until a smooth batter forms. Gently fold in chopped walnuts for added texture and nutty flavor. Heat a griddle or skillet over medium heat and ladle the pancake batter onto the surface. Cook until bubbles form on the surface, then flip and cook until golden brown. Serve the pancakes warm with maple syrup and extra banana slices on top.

These breakfast delights are just the beginning of your lacto-vegetarian culinary adventure. Stay tuned for more delicious recipes to fuel your day and nourish your body from morning till night.

Creamy Berry Smoothie Bowl

Indulge in a refreshing and nutritious start to your day with this delightful creamy berry smoothie bowl. Packed with antioxidants, vitamins, and minerals, this vibrant dish is a perfect way to fuel your body and satisfy your taste buds. Here's how to whip up this delicious breakfast treat:

Ingredients:
- 1 cup mixed frozen berries (such as strawberries, blueberries, raspberries)
- 1 ripe banana, peeled and sliced
- 1/2 cup Greek yogurt
- 1/4 cup milk (dairy or plant-based)
- Toppings of your choice: granola, sliced fresh fruit, nuts, seeds, shredded coconut, honey, or maple syrup

Instructions:

1. Blend: In a blender, combine the mixed frozen berries, sliced banana, Greek yogurt, and milk. Blend until smooth and creamy, adding more milk as needed to reach your desired consistency.

2. Pour: Once the smoothie is blended to perfection, pour it into a bowl.

3. Top: Get creative with your toppings! Sprinkle your smoothie bowl with your favorite toppings such as crunchy granola, sliced fresh fruit, nuts, seeds, shredded coconut, or a drizzle of honey or maple syrup for added sweetness.

4. Enjoy: Grab a spoon and dig in! Enjoy the creamy texture and burst of fruity flavor with every bite. Take a moment to savor the deliciousness of your homemade creamy berry smoothie bowl.

This creamy berry smoothie bowl is not only delicious but also incredibly versatile. Feel free to customize it with your favorite fruits, toppings, and add-ins to suit your taste preferences. Whether enjoyed as a quick breakfast on busy mornings or as a leisurely weekend treat, this creamy berry smoothie bowl is sure to brighten your day and leave you feeling energized and satisfied.

Veggie Omelette with Feta Cheese

Start your day with a burst of flavor and protein by treating yourself to a delicious veggie omelette with creamy feta cheese. This hearty and nutritious breakfast is a perfect way to fuel your body and satisfy your taste buds. Here's how to whip up this delightful dish:

Ingredients:
- 2 eggs
- 2 tablespoons milk
- Salt and pepper, to taste
- 1/4 cup bell peppers, diced (any color)
- 1/4 cup spinach, chopped
- 2 tablespoons red onion, finely chopped

- 2 tablespoons crumbled feta cheese

- 1 tablespoon olive oil or butter

Instructions:

1. Prep Veggies: Start by preparing your vegetables. Dice the bell peppers, chop the spinach, and finely chop the red onion. Set aside.

2. Whisk Eggs: In a mixing bowl, crack the eggs and add the milk. Season with salt and pepper, then whisk until well combined and slightly frothy.

3. Sauté Vegetables: Heat the olive oil or butter in a non-stick skillet over medium heat. Add the diced bell peppers, chopped spinach, and chopped red onion to the skillet. Sauté for 2-3 minutes, or until the vegetables are tender.

4. Pour Eggs: Once the vegetables are cooked, pour the whisked eggs into the skillet, making sure they cover the entire surface evenly.

5. Add Feta Cheese: Sprinkle the crumbled feta cheese evenly over one half of the omelette.

6. Fold and Cook: Using a spatula, carefully fold the other half of the omelette over the side with the feta cheese. Cook for an additional 1-2 minutes, or until the eggs are fully cooked and the cheese is melted.

7. Serve: Slide the omelette onto a plate and serve hot. Garnish with additional crumbled feta cheese, if desired, and fresh herbs for extra flavor.

8. Enjoy: Grab a fork and dive into this savory and satisfying veggie omelette with creamy feta cheese. Enjoy the combination of tender vegetables, fluffy eggs, and tangy feta cheese in every bite.

This veggie omelette with feta cheese is not only delicious but also incredibly versatile. Feel free to customize it with your favorite vegetables, herbs, and cheeses to suit your taste preferences. Whether enjoyed as a quick breakfast on busy mornings or as a leisurely weekend brunch, this veggie omelette is sure to brighten your day and leave you feeling satisfied and ready to tackle whatever comes your way.

Banana Walnut Pancakes

Treat yourself to a stack of fluffy and flavorful banana walnut pancakes for a delightful breakfast that's both comforting and nutritious. These pancakes are infused with the sweet aroma of ripe bananas and the satisfying crunch of toasted walnuts, making them a perfect morning indulgence. Here's how to whip up this scrumptious breakfast treat:

Ingredients:
- 1 ripe banana, mashed
- 1 cup all-purpose flour
- 1 tablespoon baking powder
- 1/4 teaspoon salt
- 1 cup milk (dairy or plant-based)
- 1 tablespoon maple syrup or honey (optional)
- 1/4 cup chopped walnuts
- Butter or cooking oil, for greasing the skillet

- Maple syrup, sliced bananas, and additional walnuts for serving

Instructions:

1. Prepare Batter: In a mixing bowl, mash the ripe banana with a fork until smooth. Add the flour, baking powder, salt, milk, and maple syrup or honey (if using) to the bowl. Stir until all the ingredients are well combined and a smooth batter forms. Fold in the chopped walnuts until evenly distributed throughout the batter.

2. Heat Skillet: Heat a non-stick skillet or griddle over medium heat. Add a small amount of butter or cooking oil to grease the surface of the skillet.

3. Cook Pancakes: Once the skillet is hot, pour about 1/4 cup of the pancake batter onto the surface for each pancake. Use the back of a spoon to spread the batter into a round shape, if needed. Cook the pancakes for 2-3 minutes, or until bubbles start to form on the surface and the edges begin to look set.

4. Flip and Cook: Carefully flip each pancake with a spatula and cook for an additional 1-2 minutes on the other side, or until golden brown and cooked through.

5. Serve: Transfer the cooked pancakes to a plate and keep them warm while you cook the remaining batter. Serve the pancakes hot, topped with maple syrup, sliced bananas, and additional chopped walnuts for extra flavor and texture.

6. Enjoy: Dive into a stack of warm and fluffy banana walnut pancakes, savoring the delicious combination of sweet bananas and crunchy walnuts in every bite. These pancakes are sure to become a favorite breakfast indulgence for lazy weekends or special occasions.

These banana walnut pancakes are not only delicious but also incredibly versatile. Feel free to customize them with your favorite toppings and add-ins, such as chocolate chips, berries, or shredded coconut, to suit your taste preferences. Whether enjoyed with a cup of hot coffee or a glass of cold milk, these pancakes are guaranteed to brighten your morning and leave you feeling satisfied and ready to take on the day ahead.

Chapter 2: Lunchtime Favorites

For a satisfying midday meal, look no further than these delectable lacto-vegetarian lunchtime favorites. From hearty salads to flavorful sandwiches, these dishes are sure to keep you fueled and energized throughout the day. Whether you're enjoying lunch at home or packing a meal to go, these recipes are both delicious and convenient.

1. Quinoa and Black Bean Salad

Whip up a nutritious and protein-packed quinoa and black bean salad for a refreshing lunch that's both satisfying and flavorful. Simply combine cooked quinoa with black beans, diced bell peppers, cherry tomatoes, corn kernels, and chopped cilantro in a large mixing bowl. Drizzle with a zesty lime vinaigrette made with olive oil, lime juice, garlic, cumin, and chili powder. Toss everything together until well combined, then chill in the refrigerator for at least 30 minutes to allow the flavors to meld.

Serve the salad cold, garnished with avocado slices and a sprinkle of crumbled feta cheese for an extra burst of flavor.

2. Caprese Sandwich with Fresh Mozzarella

Indulge in a classic Caprese sandwich featuring layers of ripe tomato, fresh mozzarella cheese, and fragrant basil leaves, drizzled with balsamic glaze and sandwiched between slices of crusty bread. To assemble the sandwich, spread a generous layer of pesto sauce on one slice of bread, then top with sliced tomatoes, mozzarella cheese, and fresh basil leaves. Drizzle with balsamic glaze and season with salt and pepper, then place another slice of bread on top to complete the sandwich. Press down gently to secure the layers, then slice the sandwich in half and enjoy immediately.

3. Spinach and Feta Stuffed Bell Peppers

For a nutritious and satisfying lunch that's as colorful as it is flavorful, try these spinach and feta stuffed bell peppers. Begin by halving bell peppers lengthwise and removing the seeds and membranes. In a mixing bowl, combine cooked quinoa, sautéed spinach, crumbled feta cheese, diced tomatoes, minced garlic, and chopped fresh herbs such as parsley or basil. Season with salt, pepper, and a pinch of red pepper flakes for added heat, then spoon the mixture into the halved bell peppers. Place the stuffed peppers on a baking sheet and bake in the oven until the peppers are tender and the filling is heated through. Serve the stuffed peppers hot, garnished with additional fresh herbs and a drizzle of balsamic glaze, if desired.

These lunchtime favorites are just a taste of the delicious and nutritious lacto-vegetarian meals you can enjoy throughout the day. Stay tuned for more mouthwatering recipes to tantalize your taste buds and inspire your culinary creativity.

Quinoa and Black Bean Salad

Elevate your lunchtime experience with a vibrant and nutritious quinoa and black bean salad. Bursting with flavor, protein, and wholesome ingredients, this salad is a perfect choice for a satisfying midday meal. Here's how to create this delightful dish:

Ingredients:

- 1 cup quinoa, rinsed
- 1 can (15 ounces) black beans, drained and rinsed
- 1 cup cherry tomatoes, halved
- 1/2 cup corn kernels (fresh, frozen, or canned)
- 1/2 cup diced bell peppers (any color)
- 1/4 cup chopped fresh cilantro
- 2 tablespoons extra virgin olive oil
- 2 tablespoons fresh lime juice
- 1 clove garlic, minced
- 1 teaspoon ground cumin
- 1/2 teaspoon chili powder
- Salt and pepper, to taste
- Avocado slices and crumbled feta cheese for garnish (optional)

Instructions:

1. Cook Quinoa: In a medium saucepan, combine the rinsed quinoa with 2 cups of water. Bring to a boil over medium-high heat, then reduce the heat to low, cover, and simmer for 15-20 minutes, or until the quinoa is tender and the water is absorbed. Remove from heat and let it cool slightly.

2. Prepare Dressing: In a small bowl, whisk together the extra virgin olive oil, lime juice, minced garlic, ground cumin, and chili powder until well combined. Season with salt and pepper to taste.

3. Combine Ingredients: In a large mixing bowl, combine the cooked quinoa, black beans, cherry tomatoes, corn kernels, diced bell peppers, and chopped cilantro. Pour the dressing over the salad and toss gently to coat all the ingredients evenly.

4. Chill: Cover the bowl and refrigerate the salad for at least 30 minutes to allow the flavors to meld and develop.

5. Serve: Once chilled, give the salad a final toss and transfer it to a serving dish. Garnish with avocado slices and crumbled feta cheese, if desired. Serve the quinoa and black bean salad as a main dish for lunch or as a side dish alongside grilled vegetables or protein.

6. Enjoy: Dive into the vibrant flavors and wholesome goodness of this quinoa and black bean salad. Each bite offers a delightful combination of tender quinoa, hearty black beans, sweet cherry tomatoes, crunchy bell peppers, and zesty dressing.

This quinoa and black bean salad is not only delicious but also incredibly versatile. Feel free to customize it with your favorite vegetables, herbs, and spices to suit your taste preferences. Whether enjoyed at home, at work, or on the go, this salad is sure to become a lunchtime favorite that you'll crave again and again.

Caprese Sandwich with Fresh Mozzarella

Transport yourself to the sunny shores of Italy with a delightful Caprese sandwich featuring creamy fresh mozzarella, ripe tomatoes, fragrant basil, and a drizzle of balsamic glaze. This classic combination of flavors is sure to satisfy your cravings for a light yet satisfying lunch. Here's how to create this delicious sandwich:

Ingredients:

- 4 slices of crusty bread (such as ciabatta or sourdough)
- 8 ounces fresh mozzarella cheese, sliced
- 2 ripe tomatoes, sliced
- Fresh basil leaves
- Balsamic glaze, for drizzling
- Pesto sauce (optional)
- Salt and pepper, to taste

Instructions:

1. Prepare Ingredients: Slice the crusty bread into thick slices, about 1/2-inch thick. Slice the fresh mozzarella cheese into thin slices. Slice the ripe tomatoes into thin rounds. Wash and dry the fresh basil leaves.

2. Assemble Sandwich: If using, spread a layer of pesto sauce on one side of each slice of bread. Arrange the sliced fresh mozzarella cheese on two slices of bread. Top the mozzarella with sliced tomatoes, overlapping them slightly. Layer the fresh basil leaves on top of the tomatoes. Season with a pinch of salt and pepper, to taste.

3. Drizzle with Balsamic Glaze: Drizzle a generous amount of balsamic glaze over the tomatoes and basil leaves. The balsamic glaze adds a tangy sweetness that complements the flavors of the sandwich perfectly.

4. Top with Bread: Place the remaining slices of bread on top of the basil leaves to complete the sandwiches.

5. Serve: Serve the Caprese sandwiches immediately, either whole or cut in half. They can be enjoyed as is or paired with a side salad or soup for a complete meal.

6. Enjoy: Sink your teeth into the layers of creamy mozzarella, juicy tomatoes, and fragrant basil, all nestled between slices of crusty bread. Each bite offers a burst of fresh flavors that will transport you to the Italian countryside.

This Caprese sandwich with fresh mozzarella is perfect for a leisurely lunch at home, a picnic in the park, or a quick bite on the go. Feel free to customize it with your favorite additions, such as avocado slices, arugula, or grilled vegetables, to make it your own. However you choose to enjoy it, this classic sandwich is sure to become a lunchtime favorite.

Spinach and Feta Stuffed Bell Peppers

Elevate your lunchtime routine with these flavorful and nutritious spinach and feta stuffed bell peppers. Packed with wholesome ingredients and bursting with savory flavors, these stuffed peppers are sure to satisfy your cravings for a satisfying midday meal. Here's how to create this delightful dish:

Ingredients:

- 4 large bell peppers (any color)
- 1 cup cooked quinoa
- 1 cup fresh spinach, chopped
- 1/2 cup crumbled feta cheese
- 1/2 cup diced tomatoes
- 2 cloves garlic, minced
- 1 tablespoon olive oil
- 1 teaspoon dried oregano
- Salt and pepper, to taste
- Fresh parsley or basil, for garnish (optional)

Instructions:

1. Prepare Bell Peppers: Preheat your oven to 375°F (190°C). Cut the tops off the bell peppers and remove the seeds and membranes from the inside. Rinse the peppers under cold water and pat them dry with paper towels. Place the peppers upright in a baking dish or on a baking sheet lined with parchment paper.

2. Prepare Filling: In a skillet, heat the olive oil over medium heat. Add the minced garlic and cook for 1-2 minutes, or until fragrant. Add the chopped spinach to the skillet and cook until wilted, about 2-3 minutes. Remove from heat and transfer the spinach to a mixing bowl. Add the cooked quinoa, diced tomatoes, crumbled feta cheese, dried oregano, salt, and pepper to the bowl. Stir until all the ingredients are well combined.

3. Stuff Bell Peppers: Divide the quinoa and spinach mixture evenly among the bell peppers, pressing down gently to pack the filling inside each pepper. Place the stuffed peppers back into the baking dish or on the baking sheet.

4. Bake: Cover the baking dish with aluminum foil and bake the stuffed peppers in the preheated oven for 25-30 minutes, or until the peppers are tender and the filling is heated through.

5. Garnish and Serve: Remove the stuffed peppers from the oven and let them cool slightly. Garnish with fresh parsley or basil, if desired, before serving. Serve the spinach and feta stuffed bell peppers hot as a satisfying lunchtime meal.

6. Enjoy: Dive into the deliciousness of these spinach and feta stuffed bell peppers, savoring the combination of tender peppers, flavorful quinoa, and creamy feta cheese with every bite.

These stuffed bell peppers are not only delicious but also incredibly versatile. Feel free to customize them with your favorite ingredients, such as diced onions, mushrooms, or olives, to suit your taste preferences. Whether enjoyed at home, at work, or on the go, these stuffed peppers are sure to become a lunchtime favorite that you'll crave again and again.

Chapter 3: Dinner Creations

Elevate your evening meals with these delectable and nutritious lacto-vegetarian dinner creations. From comforting pasta dishes to hearty casseroles, these recipes are sure to please your palate and satisfy your hunger. Whether you're cooking for one or preparing a meal for the whole family, these dinner creations are both delicious and easy to make.

1. Creamy Mushroom and Spinach Pasta

Indulge in a bowl of creamy mushroom and spinach pasta for a comforting and satisfying dinner that's ready in no time. Start by cooking your favorite pasta according to the package instructions. In a separate skillet, sauté sliced mushrooms in olive oil until they are golden brown and tender. Add minced garlic and cook for another minute, then add fresh spinach and cook until wilted. Stir in a dollop of cream cheese and a splash of milk to create a creamy sauce. Toss the cooked pasta with the mushroom and spinach mixture, season with salt and pepper, and serve hot, garnished with grated Parmesan cheese.

2. Lentil and Sweet Potato Shepherd's Pie

Warm up with a hearty lentil and sweet potato shepherd's pie that's both comforting and nutritious. Start by cooking lentils until they are tender, then sauté diced onions, carrots, and celery in a skillet until they are soft. Add cooked lentils, diced tomatoes, vegetable broth, and your favorite seasonings to the skillet and simmer until the flavors have melded together. In a separate pot, boil sweet potatoes until they are soft, then mash them with a bit of butter and milk until smooth. Spread the lentil mixture in a baking dish and top with the mashed sweet potatoes. Bake in the oven until the sweet potatoes are golden brown and the filling is bubbly. Serve hot, garnished with fresh herbs.

3. Vegetable and Chickpea Coconut Curry

Transport your taste buds to the exotic flavors of India with a vegetable and chickpea coconut curry. In a large skillet, sauté diced onions, bell peppers, and carrots until they are soft. Add minced garlic, grated ginger, and your favorite curry spices, such as cumin, coriander, turmeric, and garam masala, and cook for another minute. Stir in coconut milk, canned chickpeas (drained and rinsed), and diced tomatoes, and simmer until the vegetables are tender and the flavors have melded together. Serve the curry hot over cooked rice or quinoa, garnished with fresh cilantro and a squeeze of lime juice.

These dinner creations are just a taste of the delicious and nutritious lacto-vegetarian meals you can enjoy at the end of the day. Stay tuned for more mouthwatering recipes to tantalize your taste buds and inspire your culinary creativity.

Creamy Mushroom Risotto

Indulge in the rich and comforting flavors of creamy mushroom risotto for a luxurious dinner that's sure to impress. This classic Italian dish is creamy, flavorful, and surprisingly simple to make. Here's how to create this delicious dinner creation:

Ingredients:

- 1 1/2 cups Arborio rice
- 4 cups vegetable broth
- 2 tablespoons olive oil
- 1 onion, finely chopped
- 2 cloves garlic, minced
- 8 ounces mushrooms (such as cremini or button), sliced
- 1/2 cup dry white wine (optional)
- 1/2 cup grated Parmesan cheese
- Salt and pepper, to taste
- Fresh parsley, for garnish

Instructions:

1. **Prepare Ingredients:** In a medium saucepan, heat the vegetable broth over low heat until it is warm. Keep it warm on the stove while you prepare the risotto.

2. **Sauté Aromatics:** In a large skillet or Dutch oven, heat the olive oil over medium heat. Add the

finely chopped onion and cook until it is soft and translucent, about 3-4 minutes. Add the minced garlic and cook for another minute, until fragrant.

3. Cook Mushrooms: Add the sliced mushrooms to the skillet and cook until they are golden brown and tender, about 5-6 minutes. Season with salt and pepper to taste.

4. Toast Rice: Add the Arborio rice to the skillet with the mushrooms and stir to coat the rice in the oil. Cook for 1-2 minutes, until the rice is slightly toasted and starts to become translucent around the edges.

5. Deglaze with Wine: If using, pour in the dry white wine and stir until it is absorbed by the rice.

6. Add Broth: Begin adding the warm vegetable broth to the skillet, one ladleful at a time, stirring constantly and allowing each addition to be absorbed before adding more. Continue this process until the rice is creamy and cooked al dente, about 20-25 minutes. You may not need to use all of the broth.

7. Finish: Once the rice is cooked to your desired consistency, stir in the grated Parmesan cheese until it is melted and creamy. Taste and adjust seasoning with salt and pepper if needed.

8. Serve: Divide the creamy mushroom risotto among serving plates or bowls. Garnish with fresh parsley and additional grated Parmesan cheese, if desired. Serve hot and enjoy!

This creamy mushroom risotto is perfect for a cozy dinner at home or for entertaining guests on special occasions. Its rich and indulgent flavors are sure to make it a favorite in your dinner rotation. Buon appetito!

Lentil Curry with Coconut Milk

Treat yourself to a flavorful and satisfying dinner with this aromatic lentil curry simmered in creamy coconut milk. Bursting with spices and wholesome ingredients, this dish is perfect for cozy evenings and gatherings with loved ones. Here's how to create this delicious dinner creation:

Ingredients:
- 1 cup dry lentils (brown or green), rinsed
- 1 tablespoon coconut oil
- 1 onion, diced
- 3 cloves garlic, minced
- 1 tablespoon fresh ginger, grated
- 1 tablespoon curry powder
- 1 teaspoon ground cumin
- 1 teaspoon ground coriander
- 1/2 teaspoon turmeric
- 1/4 teaspoon cayenne pepper (optional, for heat)
- 1 can (14 ounces) diced tomatoes
- 1 can (14 ounces) coconut milk
- 2 cups vegetable broth

- 2 cups fresh spinach, chopped

- Salt and pepper, to taste

- Cooked rice or naan bread, for serving

- Fresh cilantro, for garnish

Instructions:

1. Cook Lentils: In a large pot, heat the coconut oil over medium heat. Add the diced onion and cook until softened and translucent, about 5 minutes. Stir in the minced garlic and grated ginger, and cook for another 1-2 minutes until fragrant.

2. Add Spices: Add the curry powder, ground cumin, ground coriander, turmeric, and cayenne pepper (if using) to the pot. Stir to coat the onion mixture in the spices and toast them for about 1 minute until fragrant.

3. Simmer: Pour in the diced tomatoes (with their juices), coconut milk, and vegetable broth. Stir to combine, then add the rinsed lentils to the pot. Bring the mixture to a boil, then reduce the heat to low and let it simmer, covered, for about 20-25 minutes, or until the lentils are tender and the curry has thickened.

4. Add Spinach: Stir in the chopped spinach and let it wilt into the curry for a couple of minutes. Season the curry with salt and pepper to taste.

5. Serve: Ladle the lentil curry into bowls and serve hot with cooked rice or warm naan bread. Garnish with fresh cilantro leaves for a pop of color and flavor.

6. Enjoy: Dive into the aromatic and comforting flavors of this lentil curry with coconut milk. The creamy texture, combined with the earthy lentils and vibrant spices, is sure to warm your soul and satisfy your taste buds.

This lentil curry with coconut milk is not only delicious but also packed with protein, fiber, and nutrients. It's a perfect meal for vegetarians and omnivores alike, and it's easy to customize with your favorite vegetables or additional spices. Enjoy this flavorful dinner creation any night of the week for a satisfying and nourishing meal.

Baked Eggplant Parmesan

Treat yourself to a classic Italian-inspired dish with this delicious and comforting baked eggplant Parmesan. Layers of crispy breaded eggplant slices, marinara sauce, and melted cheese come together to create a flavorful and satisfying meal. Here's how to make this dinner creation:

Ingredients:

- 2 large eggplants, sliced into 1/2-inch rounds
- Salt
- 1 cup all-purpose flour
- 3 large eggs, beaten
- 2 cups breadcrumbs (Italian seasoned breadcrumbs work well)
- 1/2 cup grated Parmesan cheese
- 2 cups marinara sauce
- 2 cups shredded mozzarella cheese
- 1/4 cup chopped fresh basil leaves, for garnish

Instructions:

1. Prep Eggplant: Place the eggplant slices on a paper towel-lined baking sheet. Sprinkle both sides of each slice with salt and let them sit for about 30 minutes. This helps to draw out excess moisture and bitterness from the eggplant. After 30 minutes, pat the eggplant slices dry with paper towels.

2. Bread Eggplant: Preheat the oven to 400°F (200°C). Set up a breading station with three shallow bowls: one with flour, one with beaten eggs, and one with breadcrumbs mixed with grated Parmesan cheese. Dip each eggplant slice into the flour, then the beaten eggs, and finally the breadcrumb mixture, pressing gently to adhere the breadcrumbs to the eggplant.

3. Bake Eggplant: Place the breaded eggplant slices on a baking sheet lined with parchment paper. Bake in the preheated oven for about 20-25 minutes, or until the eggplant is tender and the breadcrumbs are golden brown and crispy.

4. Assemble Parmesan: In a 9x13-inch baking dish, spread a thin layer of marinara sauce on the bottom. Arrange a layer of baked eggplant slices on top of the sauce, overlapping slightly. Spoon more marinara sauce over the eggplant slices, then sprinkle with shredded mozzarella cheese. Repeat the layers until all the eggplant slices are used, finishing with a layer of marinara sauce and shredded mozzarella cheese on top.

5. Bake Again: Cover the baking dish with aluminum foil and bake in the preheated oven for about 25-30 minutes, or until the cheese is melted and bubbly.

6. Serve: Remove the foil and let the baked eggplant Parmesan cool for a few minutes. Sprinkle with chopped fresh basil leaves before serving. Serve hot and enjoy!

This baked eggplant Parmesan is a comforting and satisfying meal that's perfect for a cozy night in. Serve it with a side of pasta or a green salad for a complete and delicious dinner.

Chapter 4: Snacks and Appetizers

Elevate your snacking experience with these delicious and satisfying lacto-vegetarian snacks and appetizers. Whether you're hosting a gathering with friends or simply looking for a tasty bite to enjoy between meals, these recipes are sure to please. From crispy vegetable fritters to creamy spinach and artichoke dip, there's something for everyone to enjoy. Let's dive in!

1. Crispy Vegetable Fritters

These crispy vegetable fritters are a flavorful and nutritious snack that's perfect for any occasion. Grated zucchini, carrots, and onions are mixed with eggs, flour, and seasonings to create a batter that's then pan-fried until golden brown and crispy. Serve these fritters with a dollop of Greek yogurt or tzatziki sauce for dipping.

2. Stuffed Mini Bell Peppers

For a colorful and vibrant appetizer, try these stuffed mini bell peppers filled with a creamy herbed cheese mixture. Simply halve mini bell peppers lengthwise and remove the seeds and membranes. Fill each pepper half with a mixture of cream cheese, goat cheese, fresh herbs, and a pinch of salt and pepper. Bake in the oven until the peppers are tender and the cheese is melted and bubbly.

3. Spinach and Artichoke Dip

Creamy spinach and artichoke dip is a classic appetizer that's always a crowd-pleaser. Combine thawed frozen spinach, chopped artichoke hearts, cream cheese, sour cream, mayonnaise, grated Parmesan cheese, minced garlic, and seasonings in a baking dish. Bake until the dip is hot and bubbly, then serve it with tortilla chips, crackers, or toasted bread for dipping.

4. Crispy Baked Chickpeas

Crispy baked chickpeas are a crunchy and addictive snack that's packed with protein and fiber. Simply toss cooked chickpeas with olive oil and your favorite seasonings, such as smoked paprika, garlic powder, cumin, and cayenne pepper. Spread the seasoned chickpeas on a baking sheet and bake in the oven until crispy and golden brown. Enjoy them on their own or sprinkle them over salads for added crunch.

5. Caprese Skewers

Caprese skewers are a simple yet elegant appetizer that's perfect for summer gatherings. Thread cherry tomatoes, fresh mozzarella balls, and fresh basil leaves onto skewers, then drizzle them with balsamic glaze and a sprinkle of salt and pepper. These bite-sized skewers are bursting with fresh flavors and make a beautiful addition to any appetizer spread.

These snacks and appetizers are sure to impress your guests and satisfy your cravings for delicious and flavorful bites. Whether you're hosting a party or simply snacking at home, these recipes are easy to make and full of flavor. Enjoy!

Greek Yogurt Dip with Fresh Veggies

Elevate your snacking experience with a creamy and flavorful Greek yogurt dip served alongside an array of fresh, crunchy vegetables. This nutritious and delicious appetizer is perfect for parties, gatherings, or simply as a satisfying midday snack. Here's how to make this simple and versatile dip:

Ingredients:
- 1 cup Greek yogurt
- 1 clove garlic, minced
- 1 tablespoon lemon juice
- 1 tablespoon extra virgin olive oil
- 1 tablespoon chopped fresh dill
- Salt and pepper, to taste
- Assorted fresh vegetables (such as carrots, cucumbers, bell peppers, cherry tomatoes, and celery), for dipping

Instructions:

1. Prepare Dip: In a mixing bowl, combine the Greek yogurt, minced garlic, lemon juice, extra virgin olive oil, and chopped fresh dill. Stir until all the ingredients are well combined. Season the dip with salt and pepper to taste. Adjust the seasoning according to your preference.

2. Chill: Cover the bowl with plastic wrap and refrigerate the dip for at least 30 minutes to allow the flavors to meld together and the dip to thicken slightly. This will also help the garlic to mellow out and infuse its flavor into the yogurt.

3. Prepare Vegetables: While the dip is chilling, wash and chop a variety of fresh vegetables into bite-sized pieces. Choose a colorful assortment of vegetables for a visually appealing presentation.

4. Serve: Transfer the chilled Greek yogurt dip to a serving bowl and arrange the prepared fresh vegetables around it. Garnish the dip with a drizzle of extra virgin olive oil and a sprinkle of fresh dill, if desired.

5. Enjoy: Dive into the creamy and tangy goodness of the Greek yogurt dip, paired with the crispness of the fresh vegetables. Each crunchy bite is a burst of flavor and nutrition, making this appetizer a hit with both kids and adults alike.

This Greek yogurt dip with fresh veggies is not only delicious but also packed with protein, calcium, and vitamins from the vegetables. It's a healthy and satisfying snack that's perfect for any occasion. Feel free to customize the dip with your favorite herbs and spices or add-ins like minced shallots or grated cucumber for extra flavor. Enjoy!

Avocado Toast with Tomato and Basil

Elevate your snacking game with a delicious and nutritious avocado toast topped with ripe tomatoes and fresh basil. This simple yet flavorful dish is perfect for any time of day, whether you're looking for a quick snack, a light lunch, or a satisfying appetizer. Here's how to make it:

Ingredients:

- 2 ripe avocados
- 4 slices of your favorite bread (such as whole grain or sourdough)
- 1 large tomato, thinly sliced
- Fresh basil leaves
- Extra virgin olive oil
- Salt and pepper, to taste
- Optional: Red pepper flakes, balsamic glaze, or crumbled feta cheese for garnish

Instructions:

1. Prepare Avocado: Cut the avocados in half, remove the pits, and scoop the flesh into a bowl. Use a fork to mash the avocado until smooth, or leave it slightly chunky if desired. Season with salt and pepper to taste.

2. Toast Bread: Toast the slices of bread until golden brown and crispy. You can toast them in a toaster, under the broiler, or in a skillet with a bit of olive oil.

3. Assemble Avocado Toast: Spread a generous amount of mashed avocado onto each slice of toasted bread. Use the back of a spoon to spread it evenly to the edges.

4. Add Toppings: Place thinly sliced tomatoes on top of the mashed avocado. Arrange fresh basil leaves on top of the tomatoes. Drizzle a little extra virgin olive oil over the avocado toast to add flavor and moisture.

5. Season: Sprinkle the avocado toast with a pinch of salt and freshly ground black pepper. If desired, you can also add a sprinkle of red pepper flakes for heat or a drizzle of balsamic glaze for sweetness.

6. Garnish: For an extra burst of flavor, garnish the avocado toast with crumbled feta cheese or additional fresh basil leaves.

7. Serve: Transfer the avocado toast to a serving platter or individual plates. Serve immediately and enjoy!

This avocado toast with tomato and basil is a delicious and satisfying snack or appetizer that's bursting with flavor and nutrients. It's perfect for any occasion, from casual get-togethers to elegant brunches. Feel free to customize it with your favorite toppings or additions, such as sliced radishes, arugula, or a drizzle of honey. Enjoy!

Crispy Baked Zucchini Fries

Satisfy your craving for crunchy snacks with these delicious and nutritious crispy baked zucchini fries. Coated in seasoned breadcrumbs and baked until golden brown and crispy, these zucchini fries are a healthier alternative to traditional fries. Serve them as a snack, appetizer, or side dish for any occasion. Here's how to make them:

Ingredients:
- 2 medium zucchini

- 1/2 cup all-purpose flour

- 2 large eggs, beaten

- 1 cup breadcrumbs (panko or regular)

- 1/4 cup grated Parmesan cheese

- 1 teaspoon garlic powder

- 1 teaspoon dried oregano

- 1/2 teaspoon paprika

- Salt and pepper, to taste

- Cooking spray or olive oil, for greasing

Instructions:

1. Preheat Oven: Preheat your oven to 425°F (220°C). Line a baking sheet with parchment paper and lightly grease it with cooking spray or olive oil.

2. Prepare Zucchini: Wash the zucchini and trim off the ends. Cut each zucchini in half lengthwise, then cut each half into thin strips resembling fries.

3. Set Up Breading Station: Set up a breading station with three shallow bowls. Place the flour in the first bowl, beaten eggs in the second bowl, and breadcrumbs mixed with grated Parmesan cheese, garlic powder, dried oregano, paprika, salt, and pepper in the third bowl.

4. Bread Zucchini Fries: Working one at a time, dredge each zucchini fry in the flour, shaking off any excess. Dip it into the beaten eggs, allowing any excess to drip off. Then coat it in the breadcrumb mixture, pressing gently to adhere the breadcrumbs to the zucchini. Place the breaded zucchini fry on the prepared baking sheet. Repeat with the remaining zucchini fries.

5. Bake: Arrange the breaded zucchini fries in a single layer on the baking sheet, making sure they are not touching each other. Lightly spray the tops of the fries with cooking spray or drizzle them with olive oil.

6. Bake: Bake the zucchini fries in the preheated oven for 20-25 minutes, or until they are golden brown and crispy, flipping them halfway through the cooking time for even browning.

7. Serve: Once the zucchini fries are done baking, remove them from the oven and let them cool slightly. Serve them hot with your favorite dipping sauce, such as marinara sauce, ranch dressing, or tzatziki.

8. Enjoy: Dive into the crispy goodness of these baked zucchini fries, enjoying the crunchy exterior and tender interior with every bite. They make a delicious and satisfying snack or appetizer that's perfect for sharing with friends and family.

These crispy baked zucchini fries are sure to become a favorite in your snack rotation. They're easy to make, full of flavor, and a great way to sneak in some extra veggies into your diet. Enjoy them as a guilt-free indulgence any time you're craving something crunchy and delicious!

Chapter 5: Sweets and Treats

Indulge your sweet tooth with these delightful lacto-vegetarian sweets and treats. From decadent desserts to wholesome snacks, these recipes are sure to satisfy your cravings for something sweet. Whether you're celebrating a special occasion or simply treating yourself, these delicious creations are perfect for any time of day. Let's explore some irresistible options:

1. Chocolate Avocado Mousse

Treat yourself to a creamy and indulgent chocolate avocado mousse that's both decadent and nutritious. Blend ripe avocados with cocoa powder, maple syrup, vanilla extract, and a pinch of salt until smooth and creamy. Chill the mousse in the refrigerator for a few hours to firm up, then serve it topped with fresh berries and a sprinkle of chopped nuts for added texture.

2. Peanut Butter Energy Balls

Satisfy your sweet cravings while fueling your body with these peanut butter energy balls. Mix together rolled oats, natural peanut butter, honey, chia seeds, and mini chocolate chips until well combined. Roll the mixture into bite-sized balls, then chill them in the refrigerator until firm. These energy balls make the perfect on-the-go snack or post-workout treat.

3. Fruit and Yogurt Parfait

Create a refreshing and satisfying fruit and yogurt parfait by layering Greek yogurt with your favorite fruits and toppings. Start with a base of creamy Greek yogurt, then add layers of fresh berries, sliced bananas, granola, and a drizzle of honey. Repeat the layers until you reach the top of your serving glass. Garnish with a few extra berries and a sprig of mint for a beautiful presentation.

4. Coconut Chia Pudding

Indulge in a creamy and tropical coconut chia pudding that's perfect for breakfast or dessert. Mix together coconut milk, chia seeds, maple syrup, and vanilla extract in a jar or bowl. Let the mixture chill in the refrigerator overnight, allowing the chia seeds to absorb the liquid and thicken into a pudding-like consistency. Serve the pudding topped with fresh fruit, shredded coconut, and a sprinkle of cinnamon for a delicious treat.

5. Baked Apples with Cinnamon and Honey

Enjoy the natural sweetness of baked apples with a sprinkle of cinnamon and a drizzle of honey for a comforting and wholesome treat. Core and slice apples into wedges, then arrange them in a baking dish. Sprinkle with ground cinnamon and drizzle with honey, then bake in the oven until tender and caramelized. Serve the baked apples warm with a dollop of Greek yogurt or a scoop of vanilla ice cream for an extra special touch.

These sweets and treats are perfect for satisfying your cravings for something sweet while nourishing your body with wholesome ingredients. Whether you're looking for a healthy snack or a decadent dessert, these recipes are sure to please your palate and leave you feeling satisfied. Enjoy!

Chocolate Chip Banana Bread

Indulge in a classic treat with a twist with this irresistible chocolate chip banana bread. Moist, tender, and bursting with sweet banana flavor and melty chocolate chips, this homemade bread is perfect for breakfast, dessert, or anytime you're craving a comforting treat. Here's how to make it:

Ingredients:
- 2 cups all-purpose flour
- 1 teaspoon baking powder
- 1/2 teaspoon baking soda
- 1/2 teaspoon salt
- 1/2 cup unsalted butter, softened
- 3/4 cup granulated sugar
- 2 large eggs
- 3 ripe bananas, mashed
- 1 teaspoon vanilla extract

- 1/2 cup plain Greek yogurt or sour cream

- 1 cup semi-sweet chocolate chips

Instructions:

1. Preheat Oven: Preheat your oven to 350°F (175°C). Grease a 9x5-inch loaf pan or line it with parchment paper for easy removal.

2. Prepare Dry Ingredients: In a medium bowl, whisk together the all-purpose flour, baking powder, baking soda, and salt until well combined. Set aside.

3. Cream Butter and Sugar: In a large mixing bowl, cream together the softened unsalted butter and granulated sugar until light and fluffy, using a hand mixer or stand mixer.

4. Add Eggs and Flavorings: Add the eggs, one at a time, beating well after each addition. Stir in the mashed bananas and vanilla extract until smooth and well combined.

5. Add Dry Ingredients Alternately with Yogurt:
Gradually add the dry ingredients to the banana mixture, alternating with the plain Greek yogurt or sour cream. Mix until just combined, being careful not to overmix.

6. Fold in Chocolate Chips: Gently fold in the semi-sweet chocolate chips until evenly distributed throughout the batter.

7. Bake: Pour the batter into the prepared loaf pan and spread it out evenly. Bake in the preheated oven for 50-60 minutes, or until a toothpick inserted into the center comes out clean or with a few moist crumbs.

8. Cool and Serve: Remove the banana bread from the oven and let it cool in the pan for 10 minutes before transferring it to a wire rack to cool completely. Once cooled, slice and serve the chocolate chip banana bread and enjoy!

This chocolate chip banana bread is best enjoyed warm, either plain or with a smear of butter or a dollop of whipped cream. It's perfect for breakfast, brunch, or dessert, and it's sure to become a favorite in your household. Feel free to customize it by adding chopped nuts, shredded coconut, or a sprinkle of cinnamon for extra flavor. Enjoy!

Berry Parfait with Greek Yogurt

Treat yourself to a delightful and refreshing berry parfait with creamy Greek yogurt, fresh berries, and a hint of sweetness. This parfait is not only delicious but also nutritious, making it a perfect guilt-free dessert or sweet snack. Here's how to make it:

Ingredients:
- 1 cup plain Greek yogurt
- 2 tablespoons honey or maple syrup (adjust to taste)
- 1 teaspoon vanilla extract

- 1 cup mixed berries (such as strawberries, blueberries, raspberries, and blackberries), washed and sliced if needed
- Granola or crushed nuts, for layering and garnish (optional)
- Fresh mint leaves, for garnish (optional)

Instructions:

1. Prepare Yogurt Mixture: In a small bowl, mix together the plain Greek yogurt, honey or maple syrup, and vanilla extract until smooth and well combined. Adjust the sweetness to your liking by adding more honey or maple syrup if desired. Set aside.

2. Assemble Parfait: Start by layering a spoonful of the yogurt mixture into the bottom of serving glasses or jars. Next, add a layer of mixed berries on top of the yogurt. Repeat the layers until the glasses are filled, ending with a layer of yogurt on top.

3. Garnish: If desired, sprinkle granola or crushed nuts over the top layer of yogurt for added texture and crunch. Garnish with fresh mint leaves for a pop of color and freshness.

4. Serve: Serve the berry parfait immediately, or cover and refrigerate until ready to serve. Enjoy it as a delicious dessert, breakfast, or snack any time of day.

5. Variations: Feel free to customize your berry parfait with additional toppings such as shredded coconut, chia seeds, sliced bananas, or a drizzle of honey or fruit compote. Get creative and make it your own!

This berry parfait with Greek yogurt is a simple yet elegant treat that's perfect for any occasion. It's light, refreshing, and bursting with the natural sweetness of fresh berries. Plus, it's packed with protein, calcium, and antioxidants, making it a healthy choice for satisfying your sweet cravings. Enjoy this delightful parfait as a guilt-free indulgence that will leave you feeling satisfied and energized.

Almond Butter Energy Bites

Satisfy your sweet cravings while fueling your body with these delicious and nutritious almond butter energy bites. Packed with protein, fiber, and healthy fats, these bite-sized treats are perfect for a quick snack or a pre-workout boost. Plus, they're easy to make and customizable to suit your taste preferences. Here's how to whip up a batch:

Ingredients:

- 1 cup old-fashioned oats
- 1/2 cup almond butter (or any nut or seed butter of your choice)
- 1/4 cup honey or maple syrup
- 1/4 cup ground flaxseed or chia seeds
- 1/4 cup chopped almonds or other nuts
- 1/4 cup mini chocolate chips (optional)
- 1 teaspoon vanilla extract
- Pinch of salt

Instructions:

1. Mix Ingredients: In a large mixing bowl, combine the old-fashioned oats, almond butter, honey or maple syrup, ground flaxseed or chia seeds, chopped almonds, mini chocolate chips (if using), vanilla extract, and a pinch of salt. Stir until all the ingredients are well combined.

2. Chill Mixture: Place the mixture in the refrigerator for about 30 minutes to firm up. Chilling the mixture will make it easier to roll into balls.

3. Roll into Balls: Once the mixture has chilled, remove it from the refrigerator. Using your hands, roll the mixture into bite-sized balls, about 1 inch in diameter. If the mixture is too sticky, you can lightly wet your hands with water to prevent sticking.

4. Optional Coating: If desired, you can roll the energy bites in shredded coconut, cocoa powder, or crushed nuts for added flavor and texture.

5. Chill: Place the energy bites on a baking sheet lined with parchment paper and chill them in the refrigerator for another 30 minutes to firm up.

6. Store: Once chilled, transfer the energy bites to an airtight container and store them in the refrigerator for up to one week. They can also be stored in the freezer for longer-term storage.

7. Enjoy: Grab a couple of almond butter energy bites whenever you need a quick pick-me-up or a satisfying snack. They're perfect for fueling your body before or after a workout, keeping you energized throughout the day, or satisfying your sweet tooth in a healthier way.

These almond butter energy bites are not only delicious but also wholesome and satisfying. They're the perfect grab-and-go snack for busy days or anytime you need a nutritious boost. Plus, you can customize them with your favorite add-ins like dried fruit, coconut flakes, or spices for endless flavor variations. Enjoy!

Chapter 6: Beverages and Refreshments

Quench your thirst and elevate your hydration game with these delicious and refreshing lacto-vegetarian beverages. From energizing smoothies to soothing herbal teas, these drinks are perfect for any time of day and any occasion. Whether you're looking for a morning pick-me-up, a post-workout refresher, or a soothing nighttime drink, we've got you covered. Let's explore some delightful options:

1. Tropical Green Smoothie

Blend up a taste of the tropics with this refreshing tropical green smoothie. Packed with nutrient-rich spinach, creamy coconut milk, tangy pineapple, and sweet banana, this smoothie is a delicious way to start your day on a healthy note. Simply blend all the ingredients until smooth and creamy, and enjoy a taste of paradise in every sip.

2. Iced Matcha Latte

Cool down and boost your energy levels with a refreshing iced matcha latte. Whisk together high-quality matcha powder with a splash of hot water until smooth and frothy, then pour it over ice and top it off with your choice of milk (such as almond milk or oat milk). Sweeten to taste with a drizzle of honey or maple syrup, and enjoy the earthy flavor and natural caffeine boost of this vibrant green beverage.

3. Watermelon Mint Agua Fresca

Stay hydrated with a refreshing watermelon mint agua fresca that's perfect for hot summer days. Blend fresh watermelon chunks with a handful of fresh mint leaves and a squeeze of lime juice until smooth, then strain the mixture through a fine mesh sieve to remove any pulp. Serve the agua fresca over ice with a sprig of mint for garnish, and enjoy the cool, hydrating goodness of this fruity drink.

4. Golden Turmeric Latte

Warm up and unwind with a comforting golden turmeric latte that's as nourishing as it is delicious. Heat up your choice of milk (such as coconut milk or cashew milk) with ground turmeric, ground ginger, cinnamon, black pepper, and a touch of honey or maple syrup until steaming hot. Froth the mixture with a handheld frother or blender, then pour it into a mug and savor the cozy, spiced flavor and vibrant golden hue.

5. Hibiscus Iced Tea

Cool off with a refreshing hibiscus iced tea that's as beautiful as it is flavorful. Steep dried hibiscus flowers in hot water until deeply colored and fragrant, then sweeten to taste with honey, agave syrup, or sugar. Chill the tea in the refrigerator until cold, then pour it over ice and garnish with a slice of lemon or orange for a tangy and refreshing beverage that's perfect for any time of day.

These beverages and refreshments are sure to keep you hydrated, energized, and satisfied all day long. Whether you're craving something fruity, creamy, or soothing, there's a delicious drink here for every taste preference. Cheers to happy sipping!

Mango Lassi

Indulge in a taste of India with this creamy and refreshing mango lassi. Made with ripe mangoes, creamy yogurt, and a hint of aromatic cardamom, this traditional drink is a delightful treat that's perfect for cooling off on a hot day or as a satisfying accompaniment to spicy Indian dishes. Here's how to make it:

Ingredients:
- 2 ripe mangoes, peeled, pitted, and diced
- 1 1/2 cups plain yogurt
- 1/2 cup milk (or more as needed for desired consistency)
- 2-3 tablespoons honey or sugar (adjust to taste)
- 1/2 teaspoon ground cardamom
- Ice cubes (optional)
- Chopped pistachios or almonds, for garnish (optional)

- Fresh mint leaves, for garnish (optional)

Instructions:

1. Prepare Mangoes: Peel the ripe mangoes and remove the flesh from the pit. Cut the mango flesh into chunks and place them in a blender or food processor.

2. Blend: Add the plain yogurt, milk, honey or sugar, and ground cardamom to the blender with the mango chunks. Blend until smooth and creamy. If the lassi is too thick, you can add more milk to reach your desired consistency.

3. Adjust Sweetness: Taste the lassi and adjust the sweetness to your liking by adding more honey or sugar if needed. Blend again until well combined.

4. Serve: Pour the mango lassi into glasses filled with ice cubes, if desired, to make it extra refreshing. Garnish with chopped pistachios or almonds and fresh mint leaves for a decorative touch.

5. Enjoy: Serve the mango lassi immediately and enjoy the creamy, fruity goodness with every sip. It's the perfect way to cool off and satisfy your sweet cravings on a hot day.

This mango lassi is not only delicious but also packed with vitamins, minerals, and probiotics from the yogurt. It's a healthier alternative to sugary beverages and a great way to enjoy the natural sweetness of ripe mangoes. Whether you're enjoying it as a refreshing drink on its own or pairing it with spicy Indian dishes like curry or biryani, mango lassi is sure to become a favorite in your beverage rotation. Cheers to happy sipping!

Iced Matcha Latte

Elevate your beverage game with a refreshing and energizing iced matcha latte. This vibrant green drink is not only delicious but also packed with antioxidants and natural caffeine, making it the perfect pick-me-up for any time of day. Whether you're looking for a refreshing summer drink or a satisfying alternative to your morning coffee, this iced matcha latte is sure to hit the spot. Here's how to make it:

Ingredients:

- 1 teaspoon matcha powder

- 2 tablespoons hot water

- 1 cup milk of your choice (such as almond milk, oat milk, or dairy milk)

- Ice cubes

- Optional sweetener (such as honey, maple syrup, or agave syrup), to taste

Instructions:

1. Prepare Matcha: In a small bowl or cup, whisk together the matcha powder and hot water until smooth and frothy. You can use a bamboo whisk (chasen) or a small whisk for this step. Make sure there are no clumps of matcha remaining.

2. Heat Milk (Optional): If you prefer a warm latte, you can heat the milk in a small saucepan over medium heat until steaming. However, for an iced latte, you can skip this step.

3. Combine Matcha and Milk: Pour the prepared matcha mixture into a glass filled with ice cubes. If you prefer a sweetened latte, you can add your desired amount of sweetener to the glass at this point.

4. Add Milk: Pour the milk of your choice over the matcha mixture and ice cubes. Leave a little room at the top of the glass to allow for stirring.

5. Stir: Use a spoon or a straw to stir the matcha and milk together until well combined and frothy.

6. Enjoy: Your iced matcha latte is now ready to enjoy! Sip slowly and savor the refreshing flavor and natural energy boost of this delicious beverage.

7. Optional Garnish: For an extra touch of elegance, you can garnish your iced matcha latte with a sprinkle of matcha powder or a drizzle of honey on top.

This iced matcha latte is not only delicious but also versatile. You can customize it to suit your taste preferences by adjusting the sweetness level or experimenting with different types of milk. Whether you're enjoying it as a refreshing drink on a hot day or as a morning pick-me-up, this iced matcha latte is sure to become a favorite in your beverage rotation. Cheers to happy sipping!

Watermelon Mint Cooler

Cool off on a hot day with the refreshing and hydrating taste of a watermelon mint cooler. This vibrant and flavorful drink combines the natural sweetness of watermelon with the refreshing aroma of fresh mint for a delightful beverage that's perfect for summer gatherings or any time you need a refreshing pick-me-up. Here's how to make it:

Ingredients:
- 4 cups cubed seedless watermelon
- 1/4 cup fresh mint leaves
- 1 tablespoon freshly squeezed lime juice
- 2 cups cold water or sparkling water
- Ice cubes
- Mint sprigs, for garnish (optional)

- Sliced lime, for garnish (optional)

Instructions:

1. Blend Watermelon and Mint: In a blender, combine the cubed watermelon and fresh mint leaves. Blend until smooth and well combined, and the mint leaves are finely chopped.

2. Strain (Optional): If desired, strain the watermelon mint mixture through a fine mesh sieve to remove any pulp and seeds. This step is optional, depending on your preference for texture.

3. Add Lime Juice: Stir in the freshly squeezed lime juice into the watermelon mint mixture. This will add a hint of citrus brightness to the drink.

4. Add Water: Pour the cold water or sparkling water into the watermelon mint mixture and stir to combine. Adjust the amount of water based on your desired level of sweetness and concentration.

5. Chill: Place the watermelon mint cooler in the refrigerator to chill for at least 1 hour, or until cold. Alternatively, you can serve it immediately over ice.

6. Serve: Pour the chilled watermelon mint cooler into glasses filled with ice cubes. Garnish each glass with a sprig of mint and a slice of lime for a decorative touch.

7. Enjoy: Sip and enjoy the refreshing and hydrating taste of the watermelon mint cooler. It's the perfect way to beat the heat and stay cool and refreshed on a hot day.

This watermelon mint cooler is not only delicious but also incredibly easy to make with just a few simple ingredients. It's naturally sweet, refreshing, and bursting with flavor, making it a hit with both kids and adults alike. Whether you're hosting a summer barbecue, lounging by the pool, or simply craving a refreshing beverage, this watermelon mint cooler is sure to hit the spot. Cheers to happy sipping!

Appendix

Here are some additional resources to help you on your lacto-vegetarian diet journey:

1. Vegetarian and Vegan Cooking Blogs: Explore popular vegetarian and vegan cooking blogs for recipe inspiration and tips on living a plant-based lifestyle.

2. Vegetarian and Vegan Cookbooks: Check out cookbooks dedicated to vegetarian and vegan cuisine for a wide range of delicious recipes.

3. Nutrition Websites: Visit reputable nutrition websites to learn more about the health benefits of a lacto-vegetarian diet and how to ensure you're meeting your nutritional needs.

4. Online Forums and Communities: Join online forums and communities dedicated to vegetarianism and veganism to connect with like-minded individuals and share experiences and tips.

5. Local Farmers' Markets: Visit local farmers' markets to explore a variety of fresh fruits, vegetables, and other vegetarian-friendly products.

6. Nutritional Supplements: Consider consulting with a healthcare provider about incorporating nutritional supplements such as vitamin B12, iron, and omega-3 fatty acids into your diet, especially if you're concerned about meeting your nutrient requirements.

Remember, the lacto-vegetarian diet is a personal choice, and it's important to find what works best for you. These resources can provide valuable information and support as you embark on your journey to living a healthy and fulfilling lacto-vegetarian lifestyle.

Ingredient Substitution Guide

Substituting ingredients is a common practice in cooking, especially when following specific dietary requirements or preferences. Here's a handy guide to help you navigate ingredient substitutions in your lacto-vegetarian cooking:

1. Meat Substitutes:

- Tofu: Firm tofu can often be used as a substitute for meat in dishes like stir-fries, curries, and sandwiches.

- Tempeh: Another soy-based product, tempeh has a firmer texture and nuttier flavor than tofu, making it a great meat alternative in dishes like tacos, burgers, and stews.

- Seitan: Made from wheat gluten, seitan has a chewy texture similar to meat, making it ideal for dishes like stir-fries, kebabs, and sandwiches.

2. Dairy Substitutes:

- Non-Dairy Milk: Options like almond milk, soy milk, coconut milk, and oat milk can be used in place of cow's milk in recipes like smoothies, baked goods, and sauces.

- Vegan Cheese: There are many varieties of vegan cheese available, made from ingredients like nuts, soy, or tapioca starch, which can be used in recipes that call for cheese.

- Dairy-Free Yogurt: Substitute dairy-free yogurt made from coconut, almond, or soy milk in recipes like smoothies, dips, and sauces.

3. Egg Substitutes:

- Flaxseed or Chia Seed Eggs: Mix 1 tablespoon of ground flaxseed or chia seeds with 3 tablespoons of water and let sit for a few minutes until thickened.

- Applesauce: Use 1/4 cup of unsweetened applesauce in place of one egg in recipes like muffins, pancakes, and cakes.

- Silken Tofu: Blend 1/4 cup of silken tofu until smooth and use it as a substitute for one egg in recipes like quiches, pies, and custards.

4. Butter Substitutes:

- Coconut Oil: Substitute coconut oil for butter in recipes like cookies, muffins, and pie crusts for a dairy-free option.

- Olive Oil: Use extra virgin olive oil in place of butter in recipes like sautés, dressings, and marinades for a healthier alternative.

5. Honey Substitutes:

- Maple Syrup: Use pure maple syrup in place of honey in recipes like dressings, marinades, and baked goods.

- Agave Nectar: Substitute agave nectar for honey in recipes like smoothies, cocktails, and desserts for a vegan-friendly option.

6. Wheat Flour Substitutes:

- Gluten-Free Flour Blends: Use gluten-free flour blends made from ingredients like rice flour, almond flour, or tapioca starch in place of wheat flour in recipes like cakes, cookies, and breads.

- Coconut Flour: Substitute coconut flour for wheat flour in recipes like pancakes, muffins, and brownies for a grain-free option.

Remember to consider the flavor, texture, and nutritional content of the substitute when making ingredient substitutions in your recipes. With a little experimentation, you can create delicious lacto-vegetarian dishes that suit your taste preferences and dietary needs.

Nutritional Information Chart

Maintaining a balanced and nutritious diet is important for overall health and well-being. Here's a helpful chart to reference the nutritional information of common lacto-vegetarian foods:

Food	Serving Size	Calories	Protein (g)	Fat (g)	Carbohydrates (g)	Fiber (g)	Calcium (%)	Iron (%)	Vitamin C (%)
Tofu	1/2 cup	94	10	5.5	2.3	1	20	13	0
Tempeh	1/2 cup	160	15	9	9	5	7	15	0
Greek Yogurt	1 cup	120	22	0	9	0	23	1	4
Milk (1% fat)	1 cup	102	8	2.4	12	0	30	1	0

Almond Milk	1 cup	60	1	2.5	8	1	45	4	0
Chickpeas (cooked)	1/2 cup	134	7	2.4	22	6	4	14	10
Lentils (cooked)	1/2 cup	115	9	0.4	20	8	3	18	8
Quinoa (cooked)	1/2 cup	111	4	1.8	19	2.5	2	15	0
Spinach (cooked)	1 cup	41	5	0.5	7	4	24	20	14
Kale (cooked)	1 cup	36	2	0.5	7	1.3	9	6	53
Broccoli (cooked)	1 cup	55	4	0.5	11	5	6	6	135
Brown Rice (cooked)	1/2 cup	108	2	0.6	22	1.8	1	4	0

Whole Wheat Bread	1 slice	69	3	1	12	2	6	5	0
Avocado	1/2 avocado	161	2	15	9	7	2	5	16
Almonds	1/4 cup	207	8	18	7	4	8	25	0
Chia Seeds	1 ounce	138	4	9	12	10	18	30	0
Flaxseeds	1 tablespoon	55	2	4.3	3	2.8	2	10	0
Peanut Butter	2 tablespoons	191	8	16	6	2	1	4	0
Hummus	2 tablespoons	50	2	4	2	1	2	2	1
Honey	1 tablespoon	64	0	0	17	0	0	0	0

| Maple Syrup | 1 tablespoon | 52 | 0 | 0 | 13 | 0 | 3 | 2 | 0 |
| Olive Oil | 1 tablespoon | 119 | 0 | 14 | 0 | 0 | 0 | 0 | 0 |

Note: Nutritional values are approximate and may vary based on factors such as brand, preparation method, and serving size.

Use this chart as a reference to help you make informed choices about the foods you consume as part of your lacto-vegetarian diet. Remember to focus on incorporating a variety of nutrient-dense foods to ensure you're meeting your nutritional needs.

Conclusion

In conclusion, the lacto-vegetarian diet offers a wealth of delicious and nutritious options for those looking to embrace a plant-based lifestyle. By focusing on dairy products along with fruits, vegetables, grains, legumes, nuts, and seeds, individuals can enjoy a diverse and satisfying array of meals while reaping the health benefits associated with a vegetarian diet.

Throughout this cookbook, we've explored a variety of recipes that showcase the versatility and flavor of lacto-vegetarian cuisine. From hearty breakfasts to satisfying dinners, refreshing beverages to delectable sweets, there's something for everyone to enjoy.

By incorporating more plant-based foods into your diet, you can not only improve your own health but also contribute to the well-being of the planet and support animal welfare. Whether you're interested in reducing your environmental footprint, improving your overall health, or simply exploring new culinary horizons, the lacto-vegetarian diet offers a delicious and sustainable approach to eating.

We hope this cookbook has inspired you to get creative in the kitchen and explore the wonderful world of lacto-vegetarian cooking. Remember to experiment, have fun, and enjoy the journey toward a healthier, more vibrant lifestyle. Here's to delicious dishes, simple meals, and living a healthy life!

Bon appétit!

Embracing the Lacto-Vegetarian Lifestyle

As we conclude this journey through the world of lacto-vegetarian cuisine, it's evident that embracing this lifestyle offers a myriad of benefits for both individuals and the planet. The lacto-vegetarian diet, which includes dairy products while abstaining from meat and fish, presents a sustainable and compassionate approach to eating that promotes health, environmental stewardship, and ethical treatment of animals.

By choosing to adopt a lacto-vegetarian lifestyle, individuals have the opportunity to nourish their bodies with nutrient-rich plant-based foods while reducing their environmental footprint. Research has shown that vegetarian diets are associated with lower rates of chronic diseases such as heart disease, diabetes, and certain types of cancer, making them a compelling choice for those seeking to improve their health and well-being.

Moreover, embracing the lacto-vegetarian lifestyle can have positive implications for the environment. Livestock agriculture is a significant contributor to greenhouse gas emissions, deforestation, and water pollution. By reducing or eliminating meat consumption, individuals can help mitigate these environmental impacts and promote sustainability for future generations.

In addition to its health and environmental benefits, the lacto-vegetarian lifestyle aligns with principles of compassion and respect for all living beings. By choosing plant-based foods over animal products, individuals can support the welfare of animals and advocate for a more humane and ethical food system.

As we've explored in this cookbook, the lacto-vegetarian diet offers a diverse and delicious array of culinary possibilities. From vibrant salads to hearty soups, satisfying entrees to indulgent desserts, there's no shortage of creative and flavorful dishes to enjoy.

Embracing the lacto-vegetarian lifestyle is a powerful way to promote health, sustainability, and compassion in our lives and in the world around us. Whether you're motivated by health concerns, environmental consciousness, or ethical considerations, transitioning to a lacto-vegetarian diet is a positive step toward a more vibrant and fulfilling way of living.

So let's continue to savor the delicious flavors, nourish our bodies with wholesome foods, and celebrate the joy of living a lacto-vegetarian lifestyle. Together, we can create a healthier, more sustainable, and more compassionate world for ourselves and future generations.

Final Tips for Your Journey

As you embark on or continue your journey with the lacto-vegetarian lifestyle, here are some final tips to keep in mind:

1. Variety is Key: Aim for a diverse diet that includes a wide range of fruits, vegetables, whole grains, legumes, nuts, seeds, and dairy products. Experiment with new ingredients and recipes to keep your meals exciting and satisfying.

2. Balance Nutritional Needs: Pay attention to your nutritional needs, ensuring you're getting an adequate intake of protein, vitamins, minerals, and essential fatty acids. Incorporate a variety of nutrient-dense foods into your meals to support overall health and well-being.

3. Plan Ahead: Take the time to plan your meals and snacks in advance to ensure you have nutritious options available throughout the week. Batch cooking and meal prepping can be helpful strategies for saving time and staying on track with your dietary goals.

4. Read Labels: When purchasing packaged or processed foods, be sure to read the ingredient labels carefully to identify any animal-derived ingredients that may be present. Look for certified vegetarian or vegan labels to ensure products meet your dietary preferences.

5. Stay Informed: Continue to educate yourself about nutrition, sustainability, and ethical considerations related to the lacto-vegetarian lifestyle. Stay up to date on current research and developments in the field to make informed choices that align with your values and goals.

6. Listen to Your Body: Pay attention to how different foods make you feel and adjust your diet accordingly. Everyone's nutritional needs and preferences are unique, so it's important to listen to your body and honor its signals.

7. Find Support: Seek out support from friends, family members, online communities, or local vegetarian and vegan groups. Connecting with others who share your dietary lifestyle can provide valuable support, encouragement, and inspiration along the way.

8. Enjoy the Journey: Finally, remember to enjoy the journey of exploring and embracing the lacto-vegetarian lifestyle. Celebrate the delicious flavors, nourishing foods, and positive impact you're making on your health, the environment, and the world around you.

With these final tips in mind, may your journey with the lacto-vegetarian lifestyle be filled with joy, fulfillment, and delicious culinary adventures. Here's to your health, happiness, and the vibrant, compassionate lifestyle you're creating for yourself and the planet.